Pocket Guide
for Technicians

Generic-Brand Name Reference

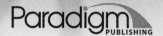

St. Paul • Los Angeles • Indianapolis

Acquisitions Editor:	Alison Brown Cerier
Developmental Editor:	Spencer Cotkin
Production Editor:	Bob Dreas
Cover and Text Designer:	Jaana Bykonich

Care has been taken to verify the accuracy of information presented in this book. However, the authors, editors, and publisher cannot accept responsibility for Web, e-mail, newsgroup, or chat room subject matter or content, or for consequences from application of the information in this book, and make no warranty, expressed or implied, with respect to its content.

Trademarks: Some of the product names and company names included in this book have been used for identification purposes only and may be trademarks or registered trade names of their respective manufacturers and sellers. The authors, editors, and publisher disclaim any affiliation, association, or connection with, or sponsorship or endorsement by, such owners.

We have made every effort to trace the ownership of all copyrighted material and to secure permission from copyright holders. In the event of any question arising as to the use of any material, we will be pleased to make the necessary corrections in future printings. Thanks are due to the aforementioned authors, publishers, and agents for permission to use the materials indicated.

ISBN 978-0-76383-481-4 (text, Study Partner CD, Pocket Guide)
ISBN 978-0-76383-480-7 (Pocket Guide)

Contents

Introduction

The *Pocket Guide for Technicians: Generic-Brand Name Reference* is provided as a supplement to *Pharmacology for Technicians, Fourth Edition,* by Don A. Ballington and Mary M. Laughlin. It is designed for quick and convenient access to drug names and includes more than 1,000 generic drugs and approximately 1,200 equivalent brand names. The drugs listed in the Pocket Guide correspond to the drugs discussed and tabulated in *Pharmacology for Technicians, Fourth Edition.* The Pocket Guide, which is sized to fit in a lab coat pocket, will be useful for students during course work and internship. Practicing health professionals also will find the Pocket Guide valuable on the job.

The 200 most commonly prescribed drugs, which are tabulated as Appendix A in *Pharmacology for Technicians, Fourth Edition*, are indicated in this Pocket Guide with an asterisk. Many instructors focus their instruction on the most commonly prescribed drugs, and this Pocket Guide can help students learn generic and brand name equivalents of these drugs.

This Pocket Guide is intended to be used only as a reference source for drug names and is not meant as a prescribing or dispensing guide.

Part I

Generic-to-Brand Drug Names

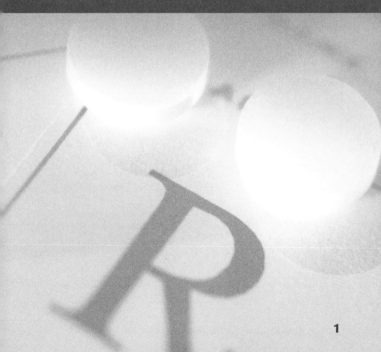

Generic Name	Brand Name
A	
abacavir	Ziagen
abarelix	Plenaxis
abatacept	Orencia
abciximab	ReoPro
acamprosate	Campral
acarbose	Precose
acebutolol	Sectral
acetaminophen*	Tylenol
acetaminophen, aspirin, caffeine	Exedrine Migraine
acetaminophen-codeine*	Phenaphen with Codeine, Tylenol with Codeine
acetazolamide	Diamox
acetylcysteine	Acetadote, Mucomyst
acitretin	Soriatane
activated carbon, charcoal	(many)
acyclovir*	Zovirax
adalimumab	Humira
adapalene	Differin
adefovir	Hepsera
albendazole	Albenza
albuterol*	Proventil, Proventil HFA, Ventolin, Ventolin HFA
alclometasone	Aclovate
aldesleukin (interleukin-2)	Proleukin
alefacept	Amevive
alemtuzumab	Campath
alendronate*	Fosamax
alfentanil	Alfenta

Generic Name	Brand Name
alfuzosin*	Uroxatral
aliskren	Tekturna
alitretinoin	Panretin
allopurinol*	Zyloprim
almotriptan	Axert
aloe gel	(many)
alprazolam*	Xanax
alprostadil	Caverject, Caverject Impulse, Edex, Muse
alteplase	Activase
altretamine	Hexalen
aluminum hydroxide	ALternaGel
aluminum hydroxide–magnesium carbonate	Gaviscon Extra Strength
aluminum hydroxide–magnesium hydroxide–simethicone	Mylanta, Mylanta Extra Strength Liquid
amantadine	Symmetrel
amcinonide	Cyclocort
amifostine	Ethyol
amikacin	(none)
amiloride	Midamor
aminoglutethimide	Cytadren
aminolevulinic acid	Levulan
aminophylline	Truphylline
amiodarone	Cordarone
amitriptyline*	Elavil
amlodipine*	Norvasc
amlodipine-atorvastatin*	Caduet
amlodipine-benazepril*	Lotrel
amlopidine-valsartan	Exforge

Generic Name	Brand Name
amobarbital	Amytal
amoxapine (TCA)	(none)
amoxicillin*	Amoxil, Trimox
amoxicillin-clavulanate*	Augmentin
amphotericin B	Abelcet (ABLC), AmBisome, Amphocin, Amphotec, Fungizone
ampicillin	Principen
ampicillin-sulbactam	Unasyn
amprenavir	Agenerase
amyl nitrite	(none)
anakinra	Kineret
anastrozole	Arimidex
anidulafungin	Eraxis
antihemophilic factor (factor VIII)	Alphanate
antipyrine-benzocaine	Auralgan
antivenin	(none)
apraclonidine	Iopidine
aprepitant	Emend
arformoterol	Brovana
aripiprazole*	Abilify
armodafinil	Nuvigil
arsenic trioxide	Trisenox
asparaginase	Elspar
aspirin (acetylsalicylic acid)	(many)
aspirin-dipyridamole*	Aggrenox
atazanavir	Reyataz
atenolol	Tenormin
atenolol-hydrochlorothiazide*	Tenoretic

Generic Name	Brand Name
atomoxetine*	Strattera
atorvastatin*	Lipitor
atovaquone-proguanil	Malarone
atracurium	Tracrium
atropine	(none)
auranofin	Ridaura
aurothioglucose	Solganal
azatadine	Optimine
azathioprine	Imuran
azelaic acid	Azelex, Finacea
azelastine	Astelin, Optivar
azithromycin*	Azasite, Zithromax, Z-PAK
aztreonam	Azactam

B

Generic Name	Brand Name
bacitracin	AK-Tracin
bacitracin-neomycin-polymyxin B	Mycitracin, Neosporin
bacitracin-neomycin-polymyxin B-hydrocortisone	Cortisporin Ointment
baclofen	Lioresal
balsalazide	Colazal
basiliximab	Simulect
becaplermin gel	Regranex
beclomethasone	Beconase AQ, QVAR, Vanceril
bedesonide-formoterol	Symbicort
benazepril*	Lotensin
benazepril-hydrochlorothiazide*	Lotensin HCT
benzalkonium chloride	Zephiran

Generic Name	Brand Name
benzocaine	Americaine, Dermoplast, Hurricaine, Orabase-B
benzonatate	Tessalon
benzoyl peroxide	Brevoxyl, Zoderm
benztropine	Cogentin
beractant	Survanta
betamethasone	Beta-Val, Diprolene, Diprosone, Luxiq
betaxolol	Betoptic, Kerlone
bethanechol	Urecholine
bevacizumab	Avastin
bicalutamide	Casodex
bimatoprost	Lumigan
bisacodyl	Dulcolax
bismuth subsalicylate	Pepto-Bismol, Kaopectate
bismuth subsalicylate–metronidazole–tetracycline	Helidac
bismuth-subcitrate potassium-metronidazole-tetracycline	Pylera
bisoprolol	Zebeta
bisoprolol-hydrochlorothiazide*	Ziac
bivalirudin	Angiomax
bleomycin	Blenoxane
bortezomib	Velcade
botulinum toxin type A	Botox
brimonidine*	Alphagan P
brinzolamide	Azopt
bromocriptine	Parlodel

Generic Name	Brand Name
budesonide*	Entocort EC, Pulmicort Respules, Pulmicort Turbuhaler, Rhinocort, Rhinecort Aqua
buffered aspirin	Ascriptin, Bufferin
bumetanide	Bumex
bupivacaine	Marcaine
buprenorphine	Buprenex, Subutex
buprenorphine-naloxone	Suboxone
bupropion*	Wellbutrin, Wellbutrin SR, Zyban
buspirone (azapirone)*	BuSpar
busulfan	Myleran
butabarbital	Butisol
butalbital-acetaminophen-caffeine	Fioricet
butalbital-aspirin-caffeine	Fiorinal
butenafine	Lotrimin Ultra, Mentax
butorphanol	Stadol, Stadol NS
C	
calcipotriene	Dovonex
calcitonin-salmon*	Miacalcin
calcium	Caltrate, Os-Cal, Tums, Viactiv
calcium carbonate–famotidine–magnesium hydroxide	Pepcid Complete
calcium carbonate-simethicone	Maalox
calcium chloride	(none)
calfactant	Infasurf
candesartan*	Atacand

Generic Name	Brand Name
capecitabine	Xeloda
capreomycin	Capastat
captopril	Capoten
carbachol	Carbastat, Miostat
carbamazepine	Epitol, Tegretol
carbamide peroxide	Gly-Oxide Oral, Debrox
carbenicillin	Geocillin
carboplatin	Paraplatin
carisoprodol*	Soma
carmustine	BiCNU
carvedilol*	Coreg
caspofungin	Cancidas
cefaclor	Ceclor
cefadroxil	Duricef
cefazolin	Ancef
cefdinir*	Omnicef
cefditoren	Spectracef
cefepime	Maxipime
cefixime	Suprax
cefotaxime	Claforan
cefpodoxime	Vantin
cefprozil*	Cefzil
ceftazidime	Fortaz
ceftibuten	Cedax
ceftizoxime	Cefizox
ceftriaxone	Rocephin
cefuroxime	Ceftin, Zinacef
celecoxib*	Celebrex
cephalexin*	Keflex
cetirizine*	Zyrtec

Generic Name	Brand Name
cetirizine-pseudoephedrine*	Zyrtec-D
cetuximab	Erbitux
cevimeline	Evoxac
chloral hydrate	(none)
chlorambucil	Leukeran
chlordiazepoxide	Librium
chlorhexidine gluconate	Hibiclens, Peridex
chloroprocaine	Nesacaine
chloroquine	Aralen
chlorpheniramine	Chlortrimeton
chlorpromazine	Thorazine
chlorpropamide	Diabinese
chlorthalidone	Hygroton
chlorzoxazone	Paraflex, Parafon Forte DSC
cholestyramine	Questran
choline magnesium trisalicylate	Trilisate
ciclesonide	Omnaris
ciclopirox	Loprox
cidofovir	Vistide
cimetidine	Tagamet, Tagamet HB
cinacalcet	Sensipar
ciprofloxacin*	Ciloxan, Cipro, Ciprodex
ciprofloxacin-dexamethasone	Ciprodex
cisatracurium	Nimbex
cisplatin	Platinol
citalopram*	Celexa
clarithromycin*	Biaxin
clemastine	Tavist Allergy
clindamycin*	Cleocin, Cleocin T

Generic Name	Brand Name
clindamycin-benzoyl peroxide	BenzaClin
clobetasol	Clobex, Olux, Temovate
clocortolone	Cloderm
clofibrate	(none)
clomipramine	Anafranil
clonazepam*	Klonopin
clonidine*	Catapres, Catapres-TTS, Duraclon
clopidogrel*	Plavix
clorazepate	Tranxene
clotrimazole	Gyne-Lotrimin, Lotrimin AF, Mycelex, Mycelex-7
clotrimazole-betamethasone*	Lotrisone
clove oil	Eugenol
clozapine	Clozaril
coal tar	Cutar, Tarsum
codeine	Codeine Contin, (various combinations)
colchicines	(none)
colesevelam	WelChol
colestipol	Colestid
colfosceril palimate	Exosurf Neonatal
conjugated estrogen*	Cenestin, Enjuvia, Premarin
conjugated estrogen-medroxyprogesterone*	Premphase, Prempro
cromolyn sodium	Crolom, Gastrocrom, Intal, Nasalcrom, Opticrom
crotamiton	Eurax
cyclobenzaprine*	Flexeril
cyclophosphamide	Cytoxan

Generic Name	Brand Name
cycloserine	Seromycin
cyclosporine	Neoral, Restasis, Sandimmune
cyproheptadine	(none)
cytarabine	Cytosar-U

D

Generic Name	Brand Name
dacarbazine	DTIC-Dome
daclizumab	Zenapax
dactinomycin	Cosmegen
dalteparin	Fragmin
danazol	Danocrine
dantrolene	Dantrium
dapsone	(none)
daptomycin	Cubicin
darbepoetin alfa	Aranesp
darifenecin	Enablex
darunavir	Prezista
dasatinib	Sprycel
daunorubicin	Cerubidine
deferoxamine	Desferal
delavirdine	Rescriptor
demeclocycline	Declomycin
denileukin diftitox	ONTAK
desflurane	Suprane
desipramine	Norpramin
desloratadine*	Clarinex
desoximetasone	Topicort
desvenlafixine	Pristiq
dexamethasone	AK-Dex, Decadron
dexmethylphenidate	Focalin

Generic Name	Brand Name
dexrazoxane	Zinecard
dextroamphetamine	Dexedrine
dextroamphetamine-amphetamine*	Adderall
dextromethorphan	Delsym
dextromethorphan-pseudoephedrine-brompheniramine	Bromfed-DM, Myphetane DX
dextrose 50%	(none)
diazepam*	Valium
diclofenac	Cataflam, Solaraze, Voltaren
diclofenac-misoprostol*	Arthrotec
dicloxacillin	(none)
didanosine	Videx
diethyl ether	Wartner
diethylpropion	Tenuate
difenoxin-atropine	Motofen
diflorasone	Florone, Psorcon
diflunisal	Dolobid
digoxin*	Lanoxicaps, Lanoxin
digoxin immune Fab	Digibind
dihydroergotamine	D.H.E. 45, Migranal
diltiazem*	Cardizem, Dilacor XR
dimercaprol, British Anti-Lewisite	BAL in Oil
dinoprostone	Cervidil, Prepidil, Prostin E
diphenhydramine	Benadryl
diphenoxylate-atropine	Lomotil
dipivefrin	Propine
dipyridamole	Persantine
dirithromycin	Dynabac

Generic Name	Brand Name
disopyramide	Norpace
disulfiram	Antabuse
divalproex*	Depakote
dobutamine	Dobutrex
docetaxel	Taxotere
docosanol	Abreva
docusate	Colace, Ex-lax Stool Softener, Surfak
docusate-senna	Senokot-S
dofetilide	Tikosyn
dolasetron	Anzemet
donepezil*	Aricept
dopamine	Intropin
doripenem	Doribax
dornase alfa	Pulmozyme
dorzolamide	Trusopt
doxazosin	Cardura
doxepin	Sinequan, Zonalon
doxorubicin	Adriamycin PFS
doxycycline*	Doryx, Vibramycin
drotrecogin alfa	Xigris
duloxetine	Cymbalta
dutasteride	Avodart
dyclonine	Cepacol Maximum Strength
E	
echothiophate iodide	Phospholine Iodide
econazole	Spectazole
edetate calcium disodium	Calcium Disodium Versenate
edrophonium	Enlon, Reversol
efalizumab	Raptiva

Generic Name	Brand Name
efavirenz	Sustiva
eflornithine	Vaniqa
eletriptan	Relpax
emtricitabine	Emtriva
enalapril*	Vasotec
enalapril-diltiazem	Teczem
enalapril-hydrochlorothiazide	Vaseretic
enflurane	Ethrane
enfuvirtide	Fuzeon
enoxaparin	Lovenox
entacapone	Comtan
entecavir	Baraclude
epinastine	Elestat
epinephrine	Adrenalin, EpiPen, Primatene Mist
epirubicin	Ellence
eplerenone	Inspra
epoetin alfa (erythropoietin)	Epogen, Procrit
epoprostenol	Flolan
eprosartan	Teveten
eptifibatide	Integrilin
ergocalciferol (vitamin D)	(none)
ergotamine	Ergomar
ergotamine-caffeine	Cafergot
erlotinib	Tarceva
ertapenem	Invanz
erythromycin	(many salts)
erythromycin	EryDerm, Ilotycin, T-Stat
erythromycin base	Eryc, Ery-Tab

Generic Name	Brand Name
erythromycin ethylsuccinate	E.E.S., EryPed
erythromycin lactobionate	Erythrocin
erythromycin stearate	Erythrocin
erythromycin-sulfisoxazole	Pediazole
escitalopram*	Lexapro
esmolol	Brevibloc
esomeprazole*	Nexium
estazolam	ProSom
estradiol*	Alora, Climara, Elestrin, Esclim, Estrace, Estraderm, Estrasorb, Estring, Evamist, Femring, Menostar, Vivelle, Vivelle Dot
estradiol cypionate-medroxyprogesterone	Lunelle
estradiol-drospirenone	Angeliq
estradiol-levonorgestrel	Climara Pro
estradiol-norethindrone	Activella, CombiPatch
estradiol-norgestimate	Ortho-Prefest
estramustine	Emcyt
estropipate	Ogen
eszopiclone*	Lunesta
etanercept	Enbrel
ethacrynic acid	Edecrin
ethambutol	Myambutol
ethinyl estradiol	Estinyl
ethinyl estradiol-desogestrel*	Cyclessa, Desogen, Kariva, Mircette, Ortho-Cept
ethinyl estradiol-drospirenone*	Yasmin, Yaz
ethinyl estradiol-ethynodiol diacetate	Demulen

Generic Name	Brand Name
ethinyl estradiol-etonogestrel	NuvaRing
ethinyl estradiol-levonorgestrel*	Aviane, Levlen, Lybrel, Nordette, Seasonale, Seasonique, Tri-Levlen, Triphasil, Trivora-28
ethinyl estradiol-norelgestromin*	Ortho Evra
ethinyl estradiol-norethindrone*	Estrostep Fe, femhrt, Loestrin Fe, Loestrin 24 Fe, Ovcon
ethinyl estradiol-norgestimate*	Ortho Tri-Cyclen, Ortho Tri-Cyclen Lo
ethinyl estradiol-norgestrel*	Lo/Ovral, Low-Ogestrel, Ovral
ethionamide	Trecator-SC
ethosuximide	Zarontin
etidronate	Didronel
etodolac	Lodine
etomidate	Amidate
etoposide	VePesid
exemestane	Aromasin
exenatide	Byetta
ezetimibe*	Zetia
ezetimbe-simvastatin*	Vytorin
F	
famciclovir	Famvir
famotidine*	Pepcid, Pepcid AC
felodipine	Plendil
fenofibrate*	TriCor
fenoldopam	Corlopam
fenoprofen	Nalfon

Generic Name	Brand Name
fentanyl*	Actiq, Duragesic, Sublimaze, Fentora, Ionsys
fentanyl-droperidol	(none)
fexofenadine*	Allegra
fexofenadine-pseudoephedrine*	Allegra-D
filgrastim	Neupogen
finasteride*	Propecia, Proscar
flavoxate	Urispas
flecainide	Tambocor
floxuridine	FUDR
fluconazole*	Diflucan
flucytosine	Ancobon
fludarabine	Fludara
flumazenil	Romazicon
flunisolide	AeroBid, Nasarel
fluocinolone	Capex, Synalar
fluocinonide	Lidex
fluorometholone	FML Forte
fluorouracil	Efudex
fluoxetine*	Prozac, Sarafem
fluphenazine	Prolixin
flurazepam	Dalmane
flurbiprofen	Ansaid, Ocufen
flutamide	Eulexin
fluticasone*	Cutivate, Flonase, Flovent
fluticasone (furoate)	Veramyst
fluticasone (propionate)	Flonase
fluticasone-salmeterol*	Advair Diskus
fluvoxamine	(none)

Generic Name	Brand Name
folic acid (vitamin B9)	(many)
fomepizole	Antizol
fomivirsen	Vitravene
fondaparinux	Arixtra
formoterol	Foradil, Perforomis
fosamprenavir	Lexiva
foscarnet	Foscavir
fosinopril	Monopril
fosphenytoin	Cerebyx
frovatriptan	Frova
fulvestrant	Faslodex
furosemide*	Lasix

G

Generic Name	Brand Name
gabapentin*	Neurontin
galantamine	Reminyl
ganciclovir	Cytovene, Vitrasert
gatifloxacin	Tequin, Zymar
gefitinib	Iressa
gemfibrozil*	Lopid
gemifloxacin	Factive
gemtuzumab	Mylotarg
gentamicin	Garamycin, Genoptic, Gentak
ginkgo	(many)
glatiramer acetate	Copaxone
glimepiride*	Amaryl
glipizide*	Glucotrol, Glucotrol XL
glipizide-metformin	Metaglip
glucagons	GlucaGen
glyburide*	DiaBeta, Glynase, Micronase
glyburide-metformin*	Glucovance

Generic Name	Brand Name
glycerin	Fleet Glycerin Suppositories
goserelin	Zoladex
granisetron	Kytril
griseofulvin	Fulvicin P/G, Fulvicin-U/F, Grifulvin V, Gris-PEG
guaifenesin*	Mucinex
guaifenesin-codeine*	Robitussin A-C
guaifenesin-dextromethorphan	Mucinex DM
guaifenesin-pseudoephedrine*	Mucinex D
guanfacine	Tenex
H	
halcinonide	Halog
halobetasol	Ultravate
haloperidol	Haldol
halothane	(none)
heparin	(none)
hexachlorophene	pHisoHex
hydralazine	Apresoline
hydrochlorothiazide (HCTZ)*	Esidrix
hydrocodone-acetaminophen*	Lortab, Lorcet, Vicodin
hydrocodone-chlorpheniramine*	Tussionex
hydrocortisone	Anusol HC, Scalpicin, Solu-Cortef
hydrocortisone butyrate	Locoid
hydrocortisone valerate	Westcort
hydrocortisone-lidocaine	Lida-Mantle HC

Generic Name	Brand Name
hydrogen peroxide	Peroxyl, (many)
hydromorphone	Dilaudid
hydroxychloroquine	Plaquenil
hydroxyurea	Hydrea
hydroxyzine	Atarax, Vistaril
hydroxyzine (antihistamine)	Vistaril
hyrdocortizone	Anusol-HC, Cortaid, Solu-Cortef

I

Generic Name	Brand Name
ibandronate*	Boniva
ibritumomab tiuxetan	Zevalin
ibuprofen*	Advil, Motrin
ibuprofen-pseudoephedrine	Advil Cold and Sinus
ibuprofen-pseudoephedrine, chlorpheniramine	Advil Allergy and Sinus
ibutilide	Corvert
idarubicin	(none)
ifosfamide	Ifex
imatinib	Gleevec
imipenem-cilastatin	Primaxin
imipramine	Tofranil
imiquimod	Aldara
immune globulin	Gamunex
indapamide	Lozol
indinavir	Crixivan
indomethacin	Indocin
infliximab	Remicade
insulin aspart	NovoLog
insulin aspart with protamine-insulin aspart	NovoLog Mix 70/30

Generic Name	Brand Name
insulin demetir	Levemir
insulin glargine*	Lantus
insulin glulsine	Apidra
insulin lispro*	Humalog
insulin lispro with protamine-insulin lispro	Humalog Mix 75/25
interferon alfa-2a	Roferon A
interferon alfa-2b	Intron A
interferon beta-1a	Avonex, Rebif
interferon beta-1b	Betaseron
ipratropium*	Atrovent
ipratropium-albuterol*	Combivent, DuoNeb
irbesartan*	Avapro
irbesartan-hydrochlorothiazide*	Avalide
irinotecan	Camptosar
iron dextran	INFeD
iron sucrose	Venofer
isoflurane	Forane
isometheptene-dichloralphenazone-acetaminophen	Midrin
isoniazid (INH)	Laniazid, Nydrazid
isoniazid-pyrazinamide-rifampin	Rifatar
isoniazid-rifampin	Rifamate
isopropl alcohol	(many)
isoproterenol	Isuprel
isosorbide dinitrate	Dilatrate-SR, Isodril
isosorbide mononitrate	Imdur, Ismo
isosorbide-hydralazine*	BiDil

Generic Name	Brand Name
isotretinoin	Accutane, Claravis
isradipine	DynaCirc
itraconazole	Sporanox
K	
kanamycin	Kantrex
ketamine	Ketalar
ketoconazole	Nizoral, Xolegel
ketoprofen	Orudis KT, Oruvail
ketorolac	Acular, Toradol
ketotifen	Zaditor
L	
labetalol	Normodyne, Trandate
lactulose	Enulose
lamivudine	Epivir, Epivir HBV
lamotrigine*	Lamictal
lansoprazole*	Prevacid
lansoprazole-amoxicillin-clarithromycin	Prevpac
lansoprazole-naproxen	Prevacid NapraPAC
latanoprost*	Xalatan
leflunomide	Arava
lepirudin	Refludan
letrozole	Femara
leucovorin	(none)
leuprolide	Eligard, Lupron Depot, Viadur
levalbuterol	Xopenex
levetiracetam	Keppra
levobupivacaine	Chirocaine
levocarnitine	Carnitor

Generic Name	Brand Name
levocetirizine	Xyzal
levodopa	Dopar
levodopa-carbidopa	Sinemet
levodopa-carbidopa-entacapone	Stalevo
levofloxacin*	Levaquin
levonorgestrel	Norplant II, Plan B
levothyroxine, T4*	Levothroid, Levoxyl, Synthroid
lidocaine	L-M-X, Solarcaine Aloe Extra Burn Relief, Xylocaine
lidocaine-diphenhydramine-Maalox	"Magic Swizzle"
lidocaine-epinephrine	Xylocaine with Epinephrine
lidocaine-prilocaine	EMLA
lindane	(none)
linezolid	Zyvox
lisdexamfetamine	Vyvanse
lisinopril*	Prinivil, Zestril
lisinopril-hydrochlorothiazide*	Zestoretic
lithium	Eskalith, Lithobid
lomustine	CeeNU
loperamide	Imodium, Imodium A-D
loracarbef	Lorabid
loratadine	Claritin
loratidine-pseudoephedrine	Claritin D
lorazepam*	Ativan
losartan*	Cozaar
losartan-hydrochlorothiazide*	Hyzaar

Generic Name	Brand Name
loteprednol	Alrex, Lotemax
lovestatin*	Mevacor
loxapine	Loxitane
lubiprostone	Amitiza
M	
mafenide	Sulfamylon
magnesium hydroxide	Phillips' Milk of Magnesia
magnesium sulfate (Epsom salts)	(none)
mannitol	Osmitrol
maprotiline	Ludiomil
maraviroc	Selzentry
mebendazole	Vermox
mechlorethamine	Mustargen
meclizine*	Antivert
meclofenamate	(none)
medroxyprogesterone	Depo-Provera, Provera
mefenamic acid	Ponstel
mefloquine	Lariam
megestrol	Megace
meloxicam*	Mobic
melphalan	Alkeran
memantine*	Namenda
meperidine	Demerol
meperidine-promethazine	Mepergan
mepivacaine	Carbocaine
meprobamate	Miltown
mequinol-tretinoin	Solage
mercaptopurine	Purinethol
meropenem	Merrem I.V.

Generic Name	Brand Name
mesalamine	Asacol, Lialda, Pentasa, Rowasa
metaproterenol	Alupent
metaxalone*	Skelaxin
metformin*	Glucophage, Riomet
methadone	Dolophine
methamphetamine	Desoxyn
methazolamide	Neptazane
methenamine	Cystex, Hiprex, Urex
methimazole	Tapazole
methocarbamol	Robaxin
methohexital	Brevital
methotrexate	Rheumatrex, Trexall
methoxy polyetherylene glycol-epoetin beta	Mircera
methyclothiazide	Enduron
methyldopa	Aldomet
methylene blue	Urolene Blue
methylergonovine	Methergine
methylphenidate*	Concerta, Daytrana, Metadate, Metadate ER, Methylin, Ritalin, Ritalin-SR
methylprednisolone*	Medrol Dose Pack, Solu-Medrol
methyltestosterone	Android, Testred
metoclopramide*	Reglan
metolazone*	Zaroxolyn
metoprolol*	Lopressor, Toprol XL
metronidazole	Flagyl, Flagyl I.V., MetroGel
mexiletine	Mexitil
micafungin	Mycamine

Generic Name	Brand Name
miconazole	Lotrimin AF, Monistat
miconazole-zinc oxide-petrolatum	Vusion
midazolam	Versed
miglitol	Glyset
milrinone	Primacor
minocycline*	Minocin
minoxidil	Loniten, Rogaine
mirtazapine*	Remeron
misoprostol	Cytotec
mitomycin	Mutamycin
mitotane	Lysodren
mitoxantrone	Novantrone
mivacurium	Mivacron
modafinil	Proigil, Sparlon
moexipril	Univasc
molindone	Moban
mometasone*	Nasonex
mometasone furoate	Elocon
montelukast*	Singulair
moricizine	Ethmozine
morphine	Astramorph/PF, Avinza, Duramorph, MS Contin
moxifloxacin*	Avelox, Vigamox
multiple vitamin complex	(many)
mupirocin*	Bactroban
muromonab-CD3	Orthoclone OKT3
mycophenolate	CellCept
mycophenolic acid	Myfortic

Generic Name	Brand Name
N	
nabumetone	Relafen
nadolol	Corgard
nafcillin	(none)
nalmefene	Revex
naloxone	Narcan
naltrexone	ReVia
naphazoline	AK-Con, Vasocon, Naphcon
naproxen*	Aleve, Anaprox, Naprosyn
naproxen-pseudoephedrine	Aleve Cold and Sinus
naratriptan	Amerge
natalizumab	Tysebri
natamycin	Natacyn
nateglinide	Starlix
nebivolol	Bystolic
nedocromil	Tilade
nefazodone	(none)
nelfinavir	Viracept
neomycin	Myciguent, Neo-Fradin
neomycin-polymyxin B	Neosporin G.U. Irrigant
neomycin-polymyxin B-dexamethasone	Maxitrol
neomycin-polymyxin B-hydrocortisone	Cortisporin Otic
neostigmine	Prostigmin
nesiritide	Natrecor
nevirapine	Viramune
niacin	Niacor
niacin-lovastatin	Advicor

Generic Name	Brand Name
niacin-simvastatin	Simcor
nicardipine	Cardene
nicotine	Commit, Habitrol, Nicoderm CQ, Nicorette, ProStep, Nicotrol
nifedipine*	Procardia
nilotinib	Tasigna
nilutamide	Nilandron
nimodipine	Nimotop
nisoldipine*	Sular
nitazoxanide	Alinia
nitrofurantoin*	Macrobid, Macrodantin
nitroglycerin*	Minitran, NitroDur, Nitrolingual, Nitrostat
nitroprusside	Nitropress
nitrous oxide (N20)	(none)
nizatidine	Axid, Axid AR
norepinephrine	Levophed
norethindrone	Micronor
norfloxacin	Noroxin
norgestrel	Ovrette
nortriptyline	Aventyl, Pamelor
NPH isophane insulin	Humulin N
NPH-regular insulin	Humulin 70/30
nystatin	Mycostatin, Nilstat

O

Generic Name	Brand Name
octreotide	Sandostatin
ofloxacin	Floxin, Ocuflox
olanzapine*	Zyprexa
olanzapine-fluoxetine	Symbyax

Generic Name	Brand Name
olmesartan*	Benicar
olopatadine*	Patanol
olsalazine	Dipentum
omalizumab	Xolair
omega-3 fatty acid	Lovaza
omeprazole*	Prilosec, Prilosec OTC
ondansetron	Zofran
orlistat	Xenical, Alli
orphenadrine	Norflex
oseltamivir	Tamiflu
oxacillin	(none)
oxaliplatin	Eloxatin
oxaprozin	Daypro
oxazepam	Serax
oxcarbazepine	Trilepta
oxiconazole	Oxistat
oxybutynin*	Ditropan, Oxytrol
oxycodone*	OxyContin
oxycodone-acetaminophen*	Endocet, Percocet, Tylox
oxycodone-aspirin	Endodan, Percodan
oxycodone-ibuprofen	Combunox
oxymetholone	Anadrol
oxymorphone	Numorphan
oxytocin	Pitocin
P	
paclitaxel	Taxol
paliperidone	Invega
palivizumab	Synagis
pancrelipase	Creon-10, Pancrease, Viokase

Generic Name	Brand Name
pancuronium	(none)
panitumumab	Vectibix
pantoprazole*	Protonix
papaverine	(none)
paregoric	(none)
paroxetine*	Paxil
pegfilgrastim	Neulasta
peginterferon alfa-2a	Pegasys
pemetrexed	Alimta
pemirolast	Alamast
penciclovir	Denavir
penicillamine	Cuprimine
penicillin G	(many), also different salts, i.e., potassium, sodium
penicillin G benzathine	Bicillin L-A
penicillin V*	Veetids
pentamidine	NebuPent, Pentam
pentazocine	Talwin
pentazocine-naloxone	Talwin NX
pentosan polysulfate sodium	Elmiron
pentoxifylline	Trental
perindopril	Aceon
permethrin	Elimite, Nix
perphenazine	Trilafon
phenazopyridine	Azo-Standard, Uristat
phenelzine	Nardil
phenobarbital	Luminal Sodium
phenol-sodium borate-sodium bicarbonate-glycerin	Ulcerease
phentermine	Adipex-P, Ionamin

Generic Name	Brand Name
phentolamine	Regitine
phenylephrine	none
phenytoin*	Dilantin
physostigmine	(none)
phytonadione	Mephyton, Vitamin K
phytonadione, vitamin K	AquaMEPHYTON
pilocarpine	Isopto Carpine, Salagen
pimecrolimus*	Elidel
pindolol	Visken
pioglitazone*	Actos
pioglitazone-metformin	Actoplus Met
piperacillin	(none)
piperacillin-tazobactam	Zosyn
pirbuterol	Maxair
piroxicam	Feldene
plicamycin	Mithracin
polyethylene glycol 3350*	GoLYTELY, HalfLytely, MiraLax
poractant alfa	Curosurf
posaconazole	Noxafil
potassium (K1+)*	Klor-Con
potassium iodide	Iosat, Lugol solution
povidone-iodine	Betadine
pralidoxime	Protopam
pramipexole	Mirapex
pramlintide	Symlin
pravastatin*	Pravachol
pravastatin-buffered aspirin	Pravigard PAC
praziquantel	Biltricide
prazosin	Minipress

Generic Name	Brand Name
prednisolone	Orapred, Pediapred
prednisone*	Deltasone
pregabalin*	Lyrica
primaquine	(none)
primidone	Mysoline
probenecid-colchicine	Col-Probenecid
procainamide	Procanbid, Pronestyl
procaine	Novocain
procarbazine	Matulane
prochlorperazine	Compazine
promethazine*	Phenergan
promethazine-codeine*	Phenergan with Codeine
promethazine-dextromethorphan	(none)
propafenone	Rythmol
propantheline	Pro-Banthine
propofol	Diprivan
propoxyphene	Darvon
propoxyphene-acetaminophen*	Darvocet-N 100
propranolol (beta blocker)*	Inderal
propylthiouracil, PTU	(none)
protamine sulfate	(none)
protriptyline	Vivactil
pseudoephedrine	Sudafed
psyllium	Fiberall, Metamucil, Perdiem Fiber Therapy
pyrantel	Pin-X
pyrazinamide	(none)
pyrethrins	Rid Mousse

Generic Name	Brand Name
pyridostigmine	Mestinon
pyridoxine, vitamin B6	(many)
Q	
quazepam	Doral
quetiapine*	Seroquel
quinapril*	Accupril
quinidine	(none)
quinine	Qualaquin
quinupristin-dalfopristin	Synercid
R	
rabeprazole*	Aciphex
radioactive iodine, 131I	(none)
raloxifene*	Evista
raltegravir	Isentress
ramelteon	Rozerem
ramipril*	Altace
ranibizumab	Lucenetis
ranitidine*	Zantac, Zantac 75
ranolozine	Ranexa
rasagiline	Azilect
regular insulin*	Humulin R
remifentanyl	Ulyiva
repaglinide	Prandin
retapamulin	Altabax
reteplase	Retavase
ribavirin	Copegus, Rebetol, Virazole
rifampin	Rifadin, Rimactane
rifapentine	Priftin
rifaximin	Xifaxan

Generic Name	Brand Name
riluzole	Rilutek
rimantadine	Flumadine
risedronate*	Actonel
risperidone*	Risperdal
ritonavir	Norvir
rituximab	Rituxan, Mabthera
rivastigmine	Exelon
rizatriptan	Maxalt, Maxalt-MLT
rocuronium	Zemuron
ropinirole*	ReQuip
rosiglitazone*	Avandia
rosiglitazone-glimepride	Avabdryl
rosiglitazone-metformin	Avandamet
rosurvastatin*	Crestor
S	
salicylate	Amigesic
salmeterol	Serevent
saquinavir	Fortovase, Invirase
sargramostim	Leukine
secobarbital	Seconal
selegiline	Eldepryl
selenium sulfide	Head & Shoulders Intensive Treatment, Selsun Blue
sertaconazole	Ertaczo
sertraline*	Zoloft
sevelamer	Renagel, Revela
sibutramine	Meridia
sildenafil*	Revatio, Viagara
silver sulfadiazine	Silvadene

Generic Name	Brand Name
simethocone	Gas Aid, Mylanta Maximum Strength, Mylicon Drops
simvastatin*	Zocor
sirolimus	Rapamune
sitagliptin	Januvia
sitagliptin-metformin	Janumet
sodium hypochlorite	Clorox
sodium nitrite	(none)
sodium phosphate	Fleet Phospho-Soda, Visicol
sodium thiosulfate	Versiclear
solfenacin	Vesicare
somatrem	Protropin
somatropin	Humatrope
sotalol	Betapace
spectinomycin	Trobicin
spironolactone*	Aldactone
stavudine	Zerit
streptomycin	(none)
streptozocin	Zanosar
succinylcholine	Quelicin
sucralfate	Carafate
sufentanil	Sufenta
sulconazole	Exelderm
sulfacetamide	Bleph-10
sulfacetamide-prednisolone	Blephamide
sulfamethoxazole-trimethoprim*	Bactrim, Bactrim DS, Cotrim, Cotrim DS, Septra, Septra DS
sulfasalazine	Azulfidine
sulfinpyrazone	Anturane

Generic Name	Brand Name
sulfisoxazole	Gantrisin
sulfur-sulfacetamide	Rosac, Rosula
sulindac	Clinoril
sumatriptan*	Imitrex
T	
tacrine	Cognex
tacrolimus	Prograf, Protopic
tadalafil*	Cialis
tamoxifen	Nolvadex
tamsulosin*	Flomax
tazarotene	Avage, Tazorac
telbivudine	Tyzeka
telithromycin	Ketek
telmisartan*	Micardis
temazepam*	Restoril
temozolomide	Temodar
tenecteplase	TNKase
tenofovir	Viread
terazosin*	Hytrin
terbinafine	Lamisil, Lamisil AT
terbutaline	Brethine
terconazole	Terazol
teriparatide	Forteo
testosterone	Androderm (nonscrotal), AndroGel, Testoderm (scrotal)
tetracaine	Cepacol Viractin, Pontocaine
tetracycline	Sumycin
theophylline	(many)
thiabendazole	Mintezol

Generic Name	Brand Name
thioguanine	Tabloid
thiopental	Pentothal
thioridazine	(none)
thiotepa	(none)
thiothixene	Navane
thyroid	Armour Thyroid
tiagabine	Gabitril
ticarcillin	Ticar
ticarcillin-clavulanate	Timentin
ticlopidine	Ticlid
tigecycline	Tygacil
tiludronate	Skelid
timolol*	Blocadren, Timoptic
tinzaparin	Innohep
tioconazole	Vagistat-1
tiotropium*	Spiriva
tipranavir	Aptivus
tirofiban	Aggrastat
tizanidine	Zanaflex
tobramycin	Nebcin, Tobrex
tobramycin-dexamethasone*	TobraDex
tocainide	Tonocard
tolbutamide	(none)
tolcapone	Tasmar
tolmetin	Tolectin
tolnaftate	Tinactin Antifungal
tolterodine*	Detrol
topiramate*	Topamax
topotecan	Hycamtin
torsemide	Demadex

Generic Name	Brand Name
tositumomab	Bexxar
tramadol*	Ultram
tramadol-acetaminophen*	Ultracet
trandolapril	Mavik
trandolapril-verapamil*	Tarka
tranylcypromine	Parnate
trastuzumab	Herceptin
travoprost	Travatan
trazodone*	Desyrel
treprostinil	Remodulin
tretinoin	Retin-A, Vesanoid, Renova
triamcinolone*	Azmacort, Kenalog, Nasacort AQ
triamterene	Dyrenium
triamterene-hydrochlorothiazide*	Dyazide, Maxzide
triazolam	Halcion
triethanolamine polypeptide-oleate condensate	Cerumenex
trifluoperazine	Stelazine
trifluridine	Viroptic
trimethobenzamide	Tigan
trimipramine	Surmontil
triprolidine-pseudoephedrine	Actifed Cold and Allergy
triptorelin	Trelstar
trospium	Sanctura
U	
unoprostone	Rescula
urea	Carmol, Keralac
urokinase	Abbokinase

Generic Name	Brand Name
ursodiol	Actigall
V	
valacyclovir*	Valtrex
valganciclovir	Valcyte
valproic acid*	Depakene
valrubicin	Valstar Preservative Free
valsartan*	Diovan
valsartan-hydrochlorothiazide*	Diovan HCT
vancomycin	Vancocin
vardenafil	Levitra
varenicline	Chantix
vasopressin	(none)
vecuronium	Norcuron
venlafaxine*	Effexor
verapamil*	Calan, Covera HS, Isoptin, Verelan
verteporfin	Visudyne
vinblastine	Velban
vincristine	Oncovin, Vincasar PFS
vitamin A	(many)
vitamin C	(many)
vitamin C-vitamin E-zinc-beta carotene	Ocuvite PreserVision
vitamin E	(many)
voriconazole	VFEND
W	
warfarin*	Coumadin
Z	
zafirlukast	Accolate

Generic Name	Brand Name
zaleplon	Sonata
zanamivir	Relenza
zidovudine, AZT	Retrovir
zileuton	Zyflo
zinc oxide	Desitin Cream
ziprasidone	Geodon
zoledronic acid	Zometa
zolmitriptan	Zomig
zolpidem*	Ambien
zonisamide	Zonegran

Part II

Brand-to-Generic
Drug Names

Brand Name	Generic Name
A	
Abbokinase	urokinase
Abelcet (ABLC)	amphotericin B
Abilify*	aripiprazole
Abreva	docosanol
Accolate	zafirlukast
Accupril*	quinapril
Accutane	isotretinoin
Aceon	perindopril
Acetadote	acetylcysteine
Aciphex*	rabeprazole
Aclovate	alclometasone
Actifed Cold and Allergy	triprolidine-pseudoephedrine
Actigall	ursodiol
Actiq*	fentanyl
Activase	alteplase
Activella	estradiol-norethindrone
Actonel*	risedronate
Actoplus Met	pioglitazone-metformin
Actos*	pioglitazone
Acular	ketorolac
Adderall*	dextroamphetamine-amphetamine
Adipex-P	phentermine
Adrenalin	epinephrine
Adriamycin PFS	doxorubicin
Advair Diskus*	fluticasone-salmeterol
Advicor	niacin-lovastatin
Advil*	ibuprofen

Brand Name	Generic Name
Advil Allergy and Sinus	ibuprofen-pseudoephedrine, chlorpheniramine
Advil Cold and Sinus	ibuprofen-pseudoephedrine
AeroBid	flunisolide
Agenerase	amprenavir
Aggrastat	tirofiban
Aggrenox*	aspirin-dipyridamole
AK-Con	naphazoline
AK-Dex	dexamethasone
AK-Tracin	bacitracin
Alamast	pemirolast
Albenza	albendazole
Aldactone*	spironolactone
Aldara	imiquimod
Aldomet	methyldopa
Aleve*	naproxen
Aleve Cold and Sinus	naproxen-pseudoephedrine
Alfenta	alfentanil
Alimta	pemetrexed
Alinia	nitazoxanide
Alkeran	melphalan
Allegra*	fexofenadine
Allegra-D*	fexofenadine-pseudoephedrine
Alli	orlistat
Alora*	estradiol
Alphagan P*	brimonidine
Alphanate	antihemophilic factor (factor VIII)
Alrex	loteprednol
Altabax	retapamulin

Brand Name	Generic Name
Altace*	ramipril
ALternaGel	aluminum hydroxide
Alupent	metaproterenol
Amaryl*	glimepiride
Ambien*	zolpidem
AmBisome	amphotericin B
Amerge	naratriptan
Americaine	benzocaine
Amevive	alefacept
Amidate	etomidate
Amigesic	salicylate
Amitiza	lubiprostone
Amoxil*	amoxicillin
Amphocin	amphotericin B
Amphotec	amphotericin B
Amytal	amobarbital
Anadrol	oxymetholone
Anafranil	clomipramine
Anaprox*	naproxen
Ancef	cefazolin
Ancobon	flucytosine
Androderm (nonscrotal)	testosterone
AndroGel	testosterone
Android	methyltestosterone
Angeliq	estradiol-drospirenone
Angiomax	bivalirudin
Ansaid	flurbiprofen
Antabuse	disulfiram
Antivert*	meclizine
Antizol	fomepizole

Brand Name	Generic Name
Anturane	sulfinpyrazone
Anusol HC	hydrocortisone
Anzemet	dolasetron
Apidra	insulin glulsine
Apresoline	hydralazine
Aptivus	tipranavir
AquaMEPHYTON	phytonadione, vitamin K
Aralen	chloroquine
Aranesp	darbepoetin alfa
Arava	leflunomide
Aricept*	donepezil
Arimidex	anastrozole
Arixtra	fondaparinux
Armour Thyroid	thyroid
Aromasin	exemestane
Arthrotec*	diclofenac-misoprostol
Asacol	mesalamine
Ascriptin	buffered aspirin
Astelin	azelastine
Astramorph/PF	morphine
Atacand*	candesartan
Atarax	hydroxyzine
Ativan*	lorazepam
Atrovent*	ipratropium
Augmentin*	amoxicillin-clavulanate
Auralgan	antipyrine-benzocaine
Avabdryl	rosiglitazone-glimepride
Avage	tazarotene
Avalide*	irbesartan-hydrochlorothiazide

Brand Name	Generic Name
Avandamet	rosiglitazone-metformin
Avandia*	rosiglitazone
Avapro*	irbesartan
Avastin	bevacizumab
Avelox*	moxifloxacin
Aventyl	nortriptyline
Aviane*	ethinyl estradiol-levonorgestrel
Avinza	morphine
Avodart	dutasteride
Avonex	interferon beta-1a
Axert	almotriptan
Axid	nizatidine
Axid AR	nizatidine
Azactam	aztreonam
Azasite*	azithromycin
Azelex	azelaic acid
Azilect	rasagiline
Azmacort*	triamcinolone
Azopt	brinzolamide
Azo-Standard	phenazopyridine
Azulfidine	sulfasalazine
B	
Bactrim*	sulfamethoxazole-trimethoprim
Bactrim DS*	sulfamethoxazole-trimethoprim
Bactroban*	mupirocin
BAL in Oil	dimercaprol, British Anti-Lewisite

Brand Name	Generic Name
Baraclude	entecavir
Beconase AQ	beclomethasone
Benadryl	diphenhydramine
Benicar*	olmesartan
BenzaClin	clindamycin-benzoyl peroxide
Betadine	povidone-iodine
Betapace	sotalol
Betaseron	interferon beta-1b
Beta-Val	betamethasone
Betoptic	betaxolol
Bexxar	tositumomab
Biaxin*	clarithromycin
Bicillin L-A	penicillin G benzathine
BiCNU	carmustine
BiDil*	isosorbide-hydralazine
Biltricide	praziquantel
Blenoxane	bleomycin
Bleph-10	sulfacetamide
Blephamide	sulfacetamide-prednisolone
Blocadren*	timolol
Boniva*	ibandronate
Botox	botulinum toxin type A
Brethine	terbutaline
Brevibloc	esmolol
Brevital	methohexital
Brevoxyl	benzoyl peroxide
Bromfed-DM	dextromethorphan-pseudoephedrine-brompheniramine

Brand Name	Generic Name
Brovana	arformoterol
Bufferin	buffered aspirin
Bumex	bumetanide
Buprenex	buprenorphine
BuSpar*	buspirone (azapirone)
Butisol	butabarbital
Byetta	exenatide
Bystolic	nebivolol
C	
Caduet*	amlodipine-atorvastatin
Cafergot	ergotamine-caffeine
Calan*	verapamil
Calcium Disodium Versenate	edetate calcium disodium
Caltrate	calcium
Campath	alemtuzumab
Campral	acamprosate
Camptosar	irinotecan
Cancidas	caspofungin
Capastat	capreomycin
Capex	fluocinolone
Capoten	captopril
Carafate	sucralfate
Carbastat	carbachol
Carbocaine	mepivacaine
Cardene	nicardipine
Cardizem*	diltiazem
Cardura	doxazosin
Carmol	urea
Carnitor	levocarnitine

Brand Name	Generic Name
Casodex	bicalutamide
Cataflam	diclofenac
Catapres*	clonidine
Catapres-TTS*	clonidine
Caverject	alprostadil
Caverject Impulse	alprostadil
Ceclor	cefaclor
Cedax	ceftibuten
CeeNU	lomustine
Cefizox	ceftizoxime
Ceftin, Zinacef	cefuroxime
Cefzil*	cefprozil
Celebrex*	celecoxib
Celexa*	citalopram
CellCept	mycophenolate
Cenestin	conjugated estrogen
Cepacol Maximum Strength	dyclonine
Cepacol Viractin	tetracaine
Cerebyx	fosphenytoin
Cerubidine	daunorubicin
Cerumenex	triethanolamine polypeptide-oleate condensate
Cervidil	dinoprostone
Chantix	varenicline
Chirocaine	levobupivacaine
Chlortrimeton	chlorpheniramine
Cialis*	tadalafil
Ciloxan*	ciprofloxacin
Cipro*	ciprofloxacin
Ciprodex	ciprofloxacin-dexamethasone

Brand Name	Generic Name
Claforan	cefotaxime
Claravis	isotretinoin
Clarinex*	desloratadine
Claritin	loratadine
Claritin D	loratidine-pseudoephedrine
Cleocin*	clindamycin
Cleocin T*	clindamycin
Climara*	estradio
Climara Pro	estradiol-levonorgestrel
Clinoril	sulindac
Clobex	clobetasol
Cloderm	clocortolone
Clorox	sodium hypochlorite
Clozaril	clozapine
Codeine Contin, (various combinations)	codeine
Cogentin	benztropine
Cognex	tacrine
Colace	docusate
Colazal	balsalazide
Colestid	colestipol
Col-Probenecid	probenecid-colchicine
CombiPatch	estradiol-norethindrone
Combivent	ipratropium-albuterol
Combunox	oxycodone-ibuprofen
Commit	nicotine
Compazine	prochlorperazine
Comtan	entacapone
Concerta*	methylphenidate
Copaxone	glatiramer acetate

Brand Name	Generic Name
Copegus	ribavirin
Cordarone	amiodarone
Coreg*	carvedilol
Corgard	nadolol
Corlopam	fenoldopam
Cortaid	hyrdocortizone
Cortisporin Ointment	bacitracin-neomycin-polymyxin B-hydrocortisone
Cortisporin Otic	neomycin-polymyxin B-hydrocortisone
Corvert	ibutilide
Cosmegen	dactinomycin
Cotrim*	sulfamethoxazole-trimethoprim
Cotrim DS*	sulfamethoxazole-trimethoprim
Coumadin*	warfarin
Covera HS*	verapamil
Cozaar*	losartan
Creon-10	pancrelipase
Crestor*	rosurvastatin
Crixivan	indinavir
Crolom	cromolyn sodium
Cubicin	daptomycin
Cuprimine	penicillamine
Curosurf	poractant alfa
Cutar	coal tar
Cutivate*	fluticasone
Cyclessa*	ethinyl estradiol-desogestrel
Cyclocort	amcinonide
Cymbalta	duloxetine

Brand Name	Generic Name
Cystex	methenamine
Cytadren	aminoglutethimide
Cytosar-U	cytarabine
Cytotec	misoprostol
Cytovene	ganciclovir
Cytoxan	cyclophosphamide

D

Brand Name	Generic Name
D.H.E. 45	dihydroergotamine
Dalmane	flurazepam
Danocrine	danazol
Dantrium	dantrolene
Darvocet-N 100*	propoxyphene-acetaminophen
Darvon	propoxyphene
Daypro	oxaprozin
Daytrana*	methylphenidate
Debrox	carbamide peroxide
Decadron	dexamethasone
Declomycin	demeclocycline
Delsym	dextromethorphan
Deltasone*	prednisone
Demadex	torsemide
Demerol	meperidine
Demulen	ethinyl estradiol-ethynodiol diacetate
Denavir	penciclovir
Depakene*	valproic acid
Depakote*	divalproex
Depo-Provera	medroxyprogesterone
Dermoplast	benzocaine

Brand Name	Generic Name
Desferal	deferoxamine
Desitin Cream	zinc oxide
Desogen*	ethinyl estradiol-desogestrel
Desoxyn	methamphetamine
Desyrel*	trazodone
Detrol*	tolterodine
Dexedrine	dextroamphetamine
DiaBeta*	glyburide
Diabinese	chlorpropamide
Diamox	acetazolamide
Didronel	etidronate
Differin	adapalene
Diflucan*	fluconazole
Digibind	digoxin immune Fab
Dilacor XR*	diltiazem
Dilantin*	phenytoin
Dilatrate-SR	isosorbide dinitrate
Dilaudid	hydromorphone
Diovan*	valsartan
Diovan HCT*	valsartan-hydrochlorothiazide
Dipentum	olsalazine
Diprivan	propofol
Diprolene	betamethasone
Diprosone	betamethasone
Ditropan*	oxybutynin
Dobutrex	dobutamine
Dolobid	diflunisal
Dolophine	methadone
Dopar	levodopa

Brand Name	Generic Name
Doral	quazepam
Doribax	doripenem
Doryx*	doxycycline
Dovonex	calcipotriene
DTIC-Dome	dacarbazine
Dulcolax	bisacodyl
DuoNeb	ipratropium-albuterol
Duraclon	clonidine
Duragesic*	fentanyl
Duramorph	morphine
Duricef	cefadroxil
Dyazide*	triamterene-hydrochlorothiazide
Dynabac	dirithromycin
DynaCirc	isradipine
Dyrenium	triamterene
E	
E.E.S.	erythromycin ethylsuccinate
Edecrin	ethacrynic acid
Edex	alprostadil
Effexor*	venlafaxine
Efudex	fluorouracil
Elavil*	amitriptyline
Eldepryl	selegiline
Elestat	epinastine
Elestrin*	estradio
Elidel*	pimecrolimus
Eligard	leuprolide
Elimite	permethrin
Ellence	epirubicin

Brand Name	Generic Name
Elmiron	pentosan polysulfate sodium
Elocon	mometasone furoate
Eloxatin	oxaliplatin
Elspar	asparaginase
Emcyt	estramustine
Emend	aprepitant
EMLA	lidocaine-prilocaine
Emtriva	emtricitabine
Enablex	darifenacin
Enbrel	etanercept
Endocet	oxycodone-acetaminophen
Endodan	oxycodone-aspirin
Enduron	methyclothiazide
Enjuvia*	conjugated estrogen
Enlon	edrophonium
Entocort EC*	budesonide
Enulose	lactulose
EpiPen	epinephrine
Epitol	carbamazepine
Epivir	lamivudine
Epivir HBV	lamivudine
Epogen	epoetin alfa (erythropoietin)
Eraxis	anidulafungin
Erbitux	cetuximab
Ergomar	ergotamine
Ertaczo	sertaconazole
Eryc	erythromycin base
EryDerm	erythromycin
EryPed	erythromycin ethylsuccinate
Ery-Tab	erythromycin base

Brand Name	Generic Name
Erythrocin	erythromycin lactobionate
Erythrocin	erythromycin stearate
Esclim*	estradiol
Esidrix*	hydrochlorothiazide (HCTZ)
Eskalith	lithium
Estinyl	ethinyl estradiol
Estrace*	estradiol
Estraderm*	estradiol
Estrasorb*	estradiol
Estring*	estradiol
Estrostep Fe	ethinyl estradiol-norethindrone
Ethmozine	moricizine
Ethrane	enflurane
Ethyol	amifostine
Eugenol	clove oil
Eulexin	flutamide
Eurax	crotamiton
Evamist*	estradiol
Evista*	raloxifene
Evoxac	cevimeline
Exedrine Migraine	acetaminophen, aspirin, caffeine
Exelderm	sulconazole
Exelon	rivastigmine
Exforge	amlopidine-valsartan
Ex-Lax Stool Softener	docusate
Exosurf Neonatal	colfosceril palimate
F	
Factive	gemifloxacin

Brand Name	Generic Name
Famvir	famciclovir
Faslodex	fulvestrant
Feldene	piroxicam
Femara	letrozole
femhrt	ethinyl estradiol-norethindrone
Femring*	estradiol
Fentora*	fentanyl
Fiberall	psyllium
Finacea	azelaic acid
Fioricet	butalbital-acetaminophen-caffeine
Fiorinal	butalbital-aspirin-caffeine
Flagyl	metronidazole
Flagyl I.V.	metronidazole
Fleet Glycerin Suppositories	glycerin
Fleet Phospho-Soda	sodium phosphate
Flexeril	cyclobenzaprine
Flolan	epoprostenol
Flomax*	tamsulosin
Flonase*	fluticasone (propionate)
Florone	diflorasone
Flovent*	fluticasone
Floxin	ofloxacin
Fludara	fludarabine
Flumadine	rimantadine
FML Forte	fluorometholone
Focalin	dexmethylphenidate
Foradil	formoterol
Forane	isoflurane

Brand Name	Generic Name
Fortaz	ceftazidime
Forteo	teriparatide
Fortovase	saquinavir
Fosamax*	alendronate
Foscavir	foscarnet
Fragmin	dalteparin
Frova	frovatriptan
FUDR	floxuridine
Fulvicin P/G	griseofulvin
Fulvicin-U/F	griseofulvin
Fungizone	amphotericin B
Fuzeon	enfuvirtide
G	
Gabitril	tiagabine
Gamunex	immune globulin
Gantrisin	sulfisoxazole
Garamycin	gentamicin
Gas Aid	simethocone
Gastrocrom	cromolyn sodium
Gaviscon Extra Strength	aluminum hydroxide–magnesium carbonate
Genoptic	gentamicin
Gentak	gentamicin
Geocillin	carbenicillin
Geodon	ziprasidone
Gleevec	imatinib
GlucaGen	glucagon
Glucophage*	metformin
Glucotrol*	glipizide
Glucotrol XL*	glipizide

Brand Name	Generic Name
Glucovance*	glyburide-metformin
Glynase*	glyburide
Gly-Oxide Oral	carbamide peroxide
Glyset	miglitol
GoLYTELY*	polyethylene glycol 3350
Grifulvin V	griseofulvin
Gris-PEG	griseofulvin
Gyne-Lotrimin	clotrimazole

H

Brand Name	Generic Name
Habitrol	nicotine
Halcion	triazolam
Haldol	haloperidol
HalfLytely*	polyethylene glycol 3350
Halog	halcinonide
Head & Shoulders Intensive Treatment	selenium sulfide
Helidac	bismuth subsalicylate–metronidazole–tetracycline
Hepsera	adefovir
Herceptin	trastuzumab
Hexalen	altretamine
Hibiclens	chlorhexidine gluconate
Hiprex	methenamine
Humalog*	insulin lispro
Humalog Mix 75/25	insulin lispro with protamine-insulin lispro
Humatrope	somatropin
Humira	adalimumab
Humulin 70/30	NPH-regular insulin
Humulin N	NPH isophane insulin

Brand Name	Generic Name
Humulin R*	regular insulin
Hurricaine	benzocaine
Hycamtin	topotecan
Hydrea	hydroxyurea
Hygroton	chlorthalidone
Hytrin*	terazosin
Hyzaar*	losartan-hydrochlorothiazide

I

Brand Name	Generic Name
Ifex	ifosfamide
Ilotycin	erythromycin
Imdur	isosorbide mononitrate
Imitrex*	sumatriptan
Imodium	loperamide
Imodium A-D	loperamide
Imuran	azathioprine
Inderal*	propranolol (beta blocker)
Indocin	indomethacin
Infasurf	calfactant
INFeD	iron dextran
Innohep	tinzaparin
Inspra	eplerenone
Intal	cromolyn sodium
Integrilin	eptifibatide
Intron A	interferon alfa-2b
Intropin	dopamine
Invanz	ertapenem
Invega	paliperidone
Invirase	saquinavir
Ionamin	phentermine
Ionsys*	fentanyl

Brand Name	Generic Name
Iopidine	apraclonidine
Iosat	potassium iodide
Iressa	gefitinib
Isentress	raltegravir
Ismo	isosorbide mononitrate
Isodril	isosorbide dinitrate
Isoptin*	verapamil
Isopto Carpine	pilocarpine
Isuprel	isoproterenol
J	
Janumet	sitagliptin-metformin
Januvia	sitagliptin
K	
Kantrex	kanamycin
Kaopectate	bismuth subsalicylate
Kariva*	ethinyl estradiol-desogestrel
Keflex*	cephalexin
Kenalog*	triamcinolone
Keppra	levetiracetam
Keralac	urea
Kerlone	betaxolol
Ketalar	ketamine
Ketek	telithromycin
Kineret	anakinra
Klonopin*	clonazepam
Klor-Con*	potassium (K^{1+})
Kytril	granisetron
L	
Lamictal*	lamotrigine

Brand Name	Generic Name
Lamisil	terbinafine
Lamisil AT	terbinafine
Laniazid	isoniazid (INH)
Lanoxicaps*	digoxin
Lanoxin*	digoxin
Lantus*	insulin glargine
Lariam	mefloquine
Lasix*	furosemide
Leukeran	chlorambucil
Leukine	sargramostim
Levaquin*	levofloxacin
Levemir	insulin demetir
Levitra	vardenafil
Levlen*	ethinyl estradiol-levonorgestrel
Levophed	norepinephrine
Levothroid*	levothyroxine, T4
Levoxyl*	levothyroxine, T4
Levulan	aminolevulinic acid
Lexapro*	escitalopram
Lexiva	fosamprenavir
Lialda	mesalamine
Librium	chlordiazepoxide
Lida-Mantle HC	hydrocortisone-lidocaine
Lidex	fluocinonide
Lioresal	baclofen
Lipitor*	atorvastatin
Lithobid	lithium
L-M-X	lidocaine
Lo/Ovral*	ethinyl estradiol-norgestrel

Brand Name	Generic Name
Locoid	hydrocortisone butyrate
Lodine	etodolac
Loestrin 24 Fe	ethinyl estradiol-norethindrone
Loestrin Fe	ethinyl estradiol-norethindrone
Lomotil	diphenoxylate-atropine
Loniten	minoxidil
Lopid*	gemfibrozil
Lopressor*	metoprolol
Loprox	ciclopirox
Lorabid	loracarbef
Lorcet*	hydrocodone-acetaminophen
Lortab*	hydrocodone-acetaminophen
Lotemax	loteprednol
Lotensin*	benazepril
Lotensin HCT*	benazepril-hydrochlorothiazide
Lotrel*	amlodipine-benazepril
Lotrimin AF	clotrimazole (cream), miconazole (powder)
Lotrimin Ultra	butenafine
Lotrisone*	clotrimazole-betamethasone
Lovaza	omega-3 fatty acid
Lovenox	enoxaparin
Low-Ogestrel*	ethinyl estradiol-norgestrel
Loxitane	loxapine
Lozol	indapamide
Lucenetis	ranibizumab

Brand Name	Generic Name
Ludiomil	maprotiline
Lugol solution	potassium iodide
Lumigan	bimatoprost
Luminal Sodium	phenobarbital
Lunelle	estradiol cypionate-medroxyprogesterone
Lunesta*	eszopiclone
Lupron Depot	leuprolide
Luxiq	betamethasone
Lybrel*	ethinyl estradiol-levonorgestrel
Lyrica*	pregabalin
Lysodren	mitotane
M	
Maalox	calcium carbonate-simethicone
Mabthera	rituximab
Macrobid*	nitrofurantoin
Macrodantin*	nitrofurantoin
"Magic Swizzle"	lidocaine-diphenhydramine-Maalox
Malarone	atovaquone-proguanil
Marcaine	bupivacaine
Matulane	procarbazine
Mavik	trandolapril
Maxair	pirbuterol
Maxalt	rizatriptan
Maxalt-MLT	rizatriptan
Maxipime	cefepime
Maxitrol	neomycin-polymyxin B-dexamethasone

Brand Name	Generic Name
Maxzide*	triamterene-hydrochlorothiazide
Medrol Dose Pack*	methylprednisolone
Megace	megestrol
Menostar*	estradio
Mentax	butenafine
Mepergan	meperidine-promethazine
Mephyton	phytonadione
Meridia	sibutramine
Merrem I.V.	meropenem
Mestinon	pyridostigmine
Metadate*	methylphenidate
Metadate ER*	methylphenidate
Metaglip	glipizide-metformin
Metamucil	psyllium
Methergine	methylergonovine
Methylin*	methylphenidate
MetroGel	metronidazole
Mevacor*	lovestatin
Mexitil	mexiletine
Miacalcin*	calcitonin-salmon
Micardis*	telmisartan
Micronase*	glyburide
Micronor	norethindrone
Midamor	amiloride
Midrin	isometheptene-dichloral-phenazone-acetaminophen
Migranal	dihydroergotamine
Miltown	meprobamate
Minipress	prazosin

Brand Name	Generic Name
Minitran*	nitroglycerin
Minocin*	minocycline
Mintezol	thiabendazole
Miostat	carbachol
MiraLax*	polyethylene glycol 3350
Mirapex	pramipexole
Mircera	methoxy polyetherylene glycol-epoetin beta
Mircette*	ethinyl estradiol-desogestrel
Mithracin	plicamycin
Mivacron	mivacurium
Moban	molindone
Mobic*	meloxicam
Monistat	miconazole
Monopril	fosinopril
Motofen	difenoxin-atropine
Motrin*	ibuprofen
MS Contin	morphine
Mucinex*	guaifenesin
Mucinex D*	guaifenesin-pseudoephedrine
Mucinex DM	guaifenesin-dextromethorphan
Mucomyst	acetylcysteine
Muse	alprostadil
Mustargen	mechlorethamine
Mutamycin	mitomycin
Myambutol	ethambutol
Mycamine	micafungin
Mycelex	clotrimazole
Mycelex-7	clotrimazole

Brand Name	Generic Name
Myciguent	neomycin
Mycitracin	bacitracin-neomycin-polmyxin B
Mycostatin	nystatin
Myfortic	mycophenolic acid
Mylanta	aluminum hydroxide–magnesium hydroxide–simethicone
Mylanta Extra Strength Liquid	aluminum hydroxide–magnesium hydroxide–simethicone
Mylanta Maximum Strength	simethocone
Myleran	busulfan
Mylicon Drops	simethocone
Mylotarg	gemtuzumab
Myphetane DX	dextromethorphan-pseudoephedrine-brompheniramine
Mysoline	primidone
N	
Nalfon	fenoprofen
Namenda*	memantine
Naphcon	naphazoline
Naprosyn*	naproxen
Narcan	naloxone
Nardil	phenelzine
Nasacort AQ*	triamcinolone
Nasalcrom	cromolyn sodium
Nasarel	flunisolide
Nasonex*	mometasone
Natacyn	natamycin

Brand Name	Generic Name
Natrecor	nesiritide
Navane	thiothixene
Nebcin	tobramycin
NebuPent	pentamidine
Neo-Fradin	neomycin
Neoral	cyclosporine
Neosporin	bacitracin-neomycin-polymyxin B
Neosporin G.U. Irrigant	neomycin-polymyxin B
Neptazane	methazolamide
Nesacaine	chloroprocaine
Neulasta	pegfilgrastim
Neupogen	filgrastim
Neurontin*	gabapentin
Nexium*	esomeprazole
Niacor	niacin
Nicoderm CQ	nicotine
Nicorette	nicotine
Nicotrol	nicotine
Nilandron	nilutamide
Nilstat	nystatin
Nimbex	cisatracurium
Nimotop	nimodipine
NitroDur*	nitroglycerin
Nitrolingual*	nitroglycerin
Nitropress	nitroprusside
Nitrostat*	nitroglycerin
Nix	permethrin
Nizoral	ketoconazole
Nolvadex	tamoxifen

Brand Name	Generic Name
Norcuron	vecuronium
Nordette*	ethinyl estradiol-levonorgestrel
Norflex	orphenadrine
Normodyne	labetalol
Noroxin	norfloxacin
Norpace	disopyramide
Norplant II, Plan B	levonorgestrel
Norpramin	desipramine
Norvasc*	amlodipine
Norvir	ritonavir
Novantrone	mitoxantrone
Novocain	procaine
NovoLog	insulin aspart
NovoLog Mix 70/30	insulin aspart with protamine-insulin aspart
Noxafil	posaconazole
Numorphan	oxymorphone
NuvaRing	ethinyl estradiol-etonogestrel
Nuvigil	armodafinil
Nydrazid	isoniazid (INH)
O	
Ocufen	flurbiprofen
Ocuflox	ofloxacin
Ocuvite PreserVision	vitamin C-vitamin E-zinc-beta carotene
Ogen	estropipate
Olux	clobetasol
Omnaris	ciclesonide
Omnicef*	cefdinir

Brand Name	Generic Name
Oncovin	vincristine
ONTAK	denileukin diftitox
Opticrom	cromolyn sodium
Optimine	azatadine
Optivar	azelastine
Orabase-B	benzocaine
Orapred	prednisolone
Orencia	abatacept
Ortho Evra	ethinyl estradiol-norelgestromin
Ortho Tri-Cyclen*	ethinyl estradiol-norgestimate
Ortho Tri-Cyclen Lo*	ethinyl estradiol-norgestimate
Ortho-Cept*	ethinyl estradiol-desogestrel
Orthoclone OKT3	muromonab-CD3
Ortho-Prefest	estradiol-norgestimate
Orudis KT	ketoprofen
Oruvail	ketoprofen
Os-Cal	calcium
Osmitrol	mannitol
Ovcon	ethinyl estradiol-norethindrone
Ovral*	ethinyl estradiol-norgestrel
Ovrette	norgestrel
Oxistat	oxiconazole
OxyContin*	oxycodone
Oxytrol*	oxybutynin
P	
Pamelor	nortriptyline
Pancrease	pancrelipase

Brand Name	Generic Name
Panretin	alitretinoin
Paraflex	chlorzoxazone
Parafon Forte DSC	chlorzoxazone
Paraplatin	carboplatin
Parlodel	bromocriptine
Parnate	tranylcypromine
Patanol*	olopatadine
Paxil*	paroxetine
Pediapred	prednisolone
Pediazole	erythromycin-sulfisoxazole
Pegasys	peginterferon alfa-2a
Pentam	pentamidine
Pentasa	mesalamine
Pentothal	thiopental
Pepcid*	famotidine
Pepcid AC*	famotidine
Pepcid Complete	calcium carbonate–famotidine–magnesium hydroxide
Pepto-Bismol	bismuth subsalicylate
Percocet	oxycodone-acetaminophen
Percodan	oxycodone-aspirin
Perdiem Fiber Therapy	psyllium
Perforomis	formoterol
Peridex	chlorhexidine gluconate
Peroxyl	hydrogen peroxide
Persantine	dipyridamole
Phenaphen with Codeine*	acetaminophen-codeine
Phenergan*	promethazine
Phenergan with Codeine*	promethazine-codeine

Brand Name	Generic Name
Phillips' Milk of Magnesia	magnesium hydroxide
pHisoHex	hexachlorophene
Phospholine Iodide	echothiophate iodide
Pin-X	pyrantel
Pitocin	oxytocin
Plaquenil	hydroxychloroquine
Platinol	cisplatin
Plavix*	clopidogrel
Plenaxis	abarelix
Plendil	felodipine
Ponstel	mefenamic acid
Pontocaine	tetracaine
Prandin	repaglinide
Pravachol*	pravastatin
Pravigard PAC	pravastatin-buffered aspirin
Precose	acarbose
Premarin*	conjugated estrogen
Premphase*	conjugated estrogen-medroxyprogesterone
Prepidil	dinoprostone
Prempro*	conjugated estrogen-medroxyprogesterone
Prevacid*	lansoprazole
Prevacid NapraPAC	lansoprazole-naproxen
Prevpac	lansoprazole-amoxicillin-clarithromycin
Prezista	darunavir
Priftin	rifapentine
Prilosec*	omeprazole
Prilosec OTC*	omeprazole

Brand Name	Generic Name
Primacor	milrinone
Primatene Mist	epinephrine
Primaxin	imipenem-cilastatin
Principen	ampicillin
Prinivil*	lisinopril
Pristiq	desvenlafixine
Pro-Banthine	propantheline
Procanbid	procainamide
Procardia*	nifedipine
Procrit	epoetin alfa (erythropoietin)
Prograf	tacrolimus
Proigil	modafinil
Proleukin	aldesleukin (interleukin-2)
Prolixin	fluphenazine
Pronestyl	procainamide
Propecia*	finasteride
Propine	dipivefrin
Proscar*	finasteride
ProSom	estazolam
ProStep	nicotine
Prostigmin	neostigmine
Prostin E	dinoprostone
Protonix*	pantoprazole
Protopam	pralidoxime
Protopic	tacrolimus
Protropin	somatrem
Proventil*	albuterol
Proventil HFA*	albuterol
Provera	medroxyprogesterone
Prozac*	fluoxetine

Brand Name	Generic Name
Psorcon	diflorasone
Pulmicort Respules*	budesonide
Pulmicort Turbuhaler*	budesonide
Pulmozyme	dornase alfa
Purinethol	mercaptopurine
Pylera	bismuth-subcitrate potassium-metronidazole-tetracycline
Q	
Qualaquin	quinine
Quelicin	succinylcholine
Questran	cholestyramine
QVAR	beclomethasone
R	
Ranexa	ranolozine
Rapamune	sirolimus
Raptiva	efalizumab
Rebetol	ribavirin
Rebif	interferon beta-1a
Refludan	lepirudin
Regitine	phentolamine
Reglan*	metoclopramide
Regranex	becaplermin gel
Relafen	nabumetone
Relenza	zanamivir
Relpax	eletriptan
Remeron*	mirtazapine
Remicade	infliximab
Reminyl	galantamine
Remodulin	treprostinil

Brand Name	Generic Name
Renagel	sevelamer
Renova	tretinoin
Renvela	sevelamer
ReoPro	abciximab
ReQuip*	ropinirole
Rescriptor	delavirdine
Rescula	unoprostone
Restasis	cyclosporine
Restoril*	temazepam
Retavase	reteplase
Retin-A	tretinoin
Retrovir	zidovudine, AZT
Revatio*	sildenafil
Reversol	edrophonium
Revex	nalmefene
ReVia	naltrexone
Reyataz	atazanavir
Rheumatrex	methotrexate
Rhinecort Aqua*	budesonide
Rhinocort*	budesonide
Rid Mousse	pyrethrins
Ridaura	auranofin
Rifadin	rifampin
Rifamate	isoniazid-rifampin
Rifatar	isoniazid-pyrazinamide-rifampin
Rilutek	riluzole
Rimactane	rifampin
Riomet*	metformin
Risperdal*	risperidone

Brand Name	Generic Name
Ritalin*	methylphenidate
Ritalin-SR*	methylphenidate
Rituxan	rituximab
Robaxin	methocarbamol
Robitussin A-C*	guaifenesin-codeine
Rocephin	ceftriaxone
Roferon A	interferon alfa-2a
Rogaine	minoxidil
Romazicon	flumazenil
Rosac	sulfur-sulfacetamide
Rosula	sulfur-sulfacetamide
Rowasa	mesalamine
Rozerem	ramelteon
Rythmol	propafenone
S	
Salagen	pilocarpine
Sanctura	trospium
Sandimmune	cyclosporine
Sandostatin	octreotide
Sarafem*	fluoxetine
Scalpicin	hyrdocortizone
Seasonale*	ethinyl estradiol-levonorgestrel
Seasonique*	ethinyl estradiol-levonorgestrel
Seconal	secobarbital
Sectral	acebutolol
Selsun Blue	selenium sulfide
Selzentry	maraviroc
Senokot-S	docusate-senna

Brand Name	Generic Name
Sensipar	cinacalcet
Septra*	sulfamethoxazole-trimethoprim
Septra DS*	sulfamethoxazole-trimethoprim
Serax	oxazepam
Serevent	salmeterol
Seromycin	cycloserine
Seroquel*	quetiapine
Silvadene	silver sulfadiazine
Simcor	niacin-simvastatin
Simulect	basiliximab
Sinemet	levodopa-carbidopa
Sinequan	doxepin
Singulair*	montelukast
Skelaxin*	metaxalone
Skelid	tiludronate
Solage	mequinol-tretinoin
Solaraze	diclofenac
Solarcaine Aloe Extra Burn Relief	lidocaine
Solganal	aurothioglucose
Solu-Cortef	hyrdocortizone
Solu-Medrol*	methylprednisolone
Soma*	carisoprodol
Sonata	zaleplon
Soriatane	acitretin
Sparlon	modafinil
Spectazole	econazole
Spectracef	cefditoren

Brand Name	Generic Name
Spiriva*	tiotropium
Sporanox	itraconazole
Sprycel	dasatinib
Stadol	butorphanol
Stadol NS	butorphanol
Stalevo	levodopa-carbidopa-entacapone
Starlix	nateglinide
Stelazine	trifluoperazine
Strattera*	atomoxetine
Sublimaze*	fentanyl
Suboxone	buprenorphine-naloxone
Subutex	buprenorphine
Sudafed	pseudoephedrine
Sufenta	sufentanil
Sular*	nisoldipine
Sulfamylon	mafenide
Sumycin	tetracycline
Suprane	desflurane
Suprax	cefixime
Surfak	docusate
Surmontil	trimipramine
Survanta	beractant
Sustiva	efavirenz
Symbicort	bedesonide-formoterol
Symbyax	olanzapine-fluoxetine
Symlin	pramlintide
Symmetrel	amantadine
Synagis	palivizumab
Synalar	fluocinolone

Brand Name	Generic Name
Synercid	quinupristin-dalfopristin
Synthroid*	levothyroxine, T4
T	
Tabloid	thioguanine
Tagamet	cimetidine
Tagamet HB	cimetidine
Talwin	pentazocine
Talwin NX	pentazocine-naloxone
Tambocor	flecainide
Tamiflu	oseltamivir
Tapazole	methimazole
Tarceva	erlotinib
Tarka*	trandolapril-verapamil
Tarsum	coal tar
Tasigna	nilotinib
Tasmar	tolcapone
Tavist Allergy	clemastine
Taxol	paclitaxel
Taxotere	docetaxel
Tazorac	tazarotene
Teczem	enalapril-diltiazem
Tegretol	carbamazepine
Tekturna	aliskren
Temodar	temozolomide
Temovate	clobetasol
Tenex	guanfacine
Tenoretic*	atenolol-chlorthalidone
Tenormin	atenolol
Tenuate	diethylpropion

Brand Name	Generic Name
Tequin	gatifloxacin
Terazol	terconazole
Tessalon	benzonatate
Testoderm (scrotal)	testosterone
Testred	methyltestosterone
Teveten	eprosartan
Thorazine	chlorpromazine
Ticar	ticarcillin
Ticlid	ticlopidine
Tigan	trimethobenzamide
Tikosyn	dofetilide
Tilade	nedocromil
Timentin	ticarcillin-clavulanate
Timoptic*	timolol
Tinactin Antifungal	tolnaftate
TNKase	tenecteplase
TobraDex*	tobramycin-dexamethasone
Tobrex	tobramycin
Tofranil	imipramine
Tolectin	tolmetin
Tonocard	tocainide
Topamax*	topiramate
Topicort	desoximetasone
Toprol XL*	metoprolol
Toradol	ketorolac
Tracrium	atracurium
Trandate	labetalol
Tranxene	clorazepate
Travatan	travoprost

Brand Name	Generic Name
Trecator-SC	ethionamide
Trelstar	triptorelin
Trental	pentoxifylline
Trexall	methotrexate
TriCor*	fenofibrate
Trilafon	perphenazine
Trilepta	oxcarbazepine
Tri-Levlen*	ethinyl estradiol-levonorgestrel
Trilisate	choline magnesium trisalicylate
Trimox*	amoxicillin
Triphasil*	ethinyl estradiol-levonorgestrel
Trisenox	arsenic trioxide
Trivora-28*	ethinyl estradiol-levonorgestrel
Trobicin	spectinomycin
Truphylline	aminophylline
Trusopt	dorzolamide
T-Stat	erythromycin
Tums	calcium
Tussionex*	hydrocodone-chlorpheniramine
Tygacil	tigecycline
Tylenol*	acetaminophen
Tylenol with Codeine	acetaminophen-codeine
Tylox	oxycodone-acetaminophen
Tysebri	natalizumab
Tyzeka	telbivudine

Brand Name	Generic Name
U	
Ulcerease	phenol-sodium borate-sodium bicarbonate-glycerin
Ultracet*	tramadol-acetaminophen
Ultram*	tramadol
Ultravate	halobetasol
Ulyiva	remifentanyl
Unasyn	ampicillin-sulbactam
Univasc	moexipril
Urecholine	bethanechol
Urex	methenamine
Urispas	flavoxate
Uristat	phenazopyridine
Urolene Blue	methylene blue
Uroxatral	alfuzosin
V	
Vagistat-1	tioconazole
Valcyte	valganciclovir
Valium*	diazepam
Valstar Preservative Free	valrubicin
Valtrex*	valacyclovir
Vanceril	beclomethasone
Vancocin	vancomycin
Vaniqa	eflornithine
Vantin	cefpodoxime
Vaseretic	enalapril-hydrochlorothiazide
Vasocon	naphazoline
Vasotec*	enalapril
Vectibix	panitumumab

Brand Name	Generic Name
Veetids*	penicillin V
Velban	vinblastine
Velcade	bortezomib
Venofer	iron sucrose
Ventolin*	albuterol
Ventolin HFA*	albuterol
VePesid	etoposide
Veramyst	fluticasone (furoate)
Verelan*	verapamil
Vermox	mebendazole
Versed	midazolam
Versiclear	sodium thiosulfate
Vesanoid	tretinoin
Vesicare	solfenacin
VFEND	voriconazole
Viactiv	calcium
Viadur	leuprolide
Viagara*	sildenafil
Vibramycin*	doxycycline
Vicodin*	hydrocodone-acetaminophen
Videx	didanosine
Vigamox*	moxifloxacin
Vincasar PFS	vincristine
Viokase	pancrelipase
Viracept	nelfinavir
Viramune	nevirapine
Virazole	ribavirin
Viread	tenofovir
Viroptic	trifluridine

Brand Name	Generic Name
Visicol	sodium phosphate
Visken	pindolol
Vistaril	hydroxyzine
Vistaril	hydroxyzine (antihistamine)
Vistide	cidofovir
Visudyne	verteporfin
Vitamin K	phytonadione
Vitrasert	ganciclovir
Vitravene	fomivirsen
Vivactil	protriptyline
Vivelle*	estradio
Vivelle Dot*	estradio
Voltaren	diclofenac
Vusion	miconazole-zinc oxide-petrolatum
Vytorin*	ezetimbe-simvastatin
Vyvanse	lisdexamfetamine
W	
Wartner	diethyl ether
WelChol	colesevelam
Wellbutrin*	bupropion
Wellbutrin SR*	bupropion
Westcort	hydrocortisone valerate
X	
Xalatan	latanoprost
Xanax	alprazolam
Xeloda	capecitabine
Xenical	orlistat
Xifaxan	rifaximin

Brand Name	Generic Name
Xigris	drotrecogin alfa
Xolair	omalizumab
Xolegel	ketoconazole
Xopenex	levalbuterol
Xylocaine	lidocaine
Xylocaine with Epinephrine	lidocaine-epinephrine
Xyzal	levocetirizine
Y	
Yasmin*	ethinyl estradiol-drospirenone
Yaz*	ethinyl estradiol-drospirenone
Z	
Zaditor	ketotifen
Zanaflex	tizanidine
Zanosar	streptozocin
Zantac*	ranitidine
Zantac 75*	ranitidine
Zarontin	ethosuximide
Zaroxolyn*	metolazone
Zebeta	bisoprolol
Zemuron	rocuronium
Zenapax	daclizumab
Zephiran	benzalkonium chloride
Zerit	stavudine
Zestoric*	lisinopril-hydrochlorothiazide
Zestril*	lisinopril
Zetia*	ezetimibe
Zevalin	ibritumomab tiuxetan

Brand Name	Generic Name
Ziac*	bisoprolol-hydrochlorothiazide
Ziagen	abacavir
Zinecard	dexrazoxane
Zithromax*	azithromycin
Zocor*	simvastatin
Zoderm	benzoyl peroxide
Zofran	ondansetron
Zoladex	goserelin
Zoloft*	sertraline
Zometa	zoledronic acid
Zomig	zolmitriptan
Zonalon	doxepin
Zonegran	zonisamide
Zosyn	piperacillin-tazobactam
Zovirax*	acyclovir
Z-PAK*	azithromycin
Zyban*	bupropion
Zyflo	zileuton
Zyloprim*	allopurinol
Zymar	gatifloxacin
Zyprexa*	olanzapine
Zyrtec*	cetirizine
Zyrtec-D*	cetirizine-pseudoephedrine
Zyvox	linezolid

Notes

Notes

Notes

Notes